Staying Alive Is Not Enough.

"I want to be living, not just existing"

By Noah Anonis.

TO THE PEOPLE OF THE WORLD WHO
CONTINUE TO FIGHT THEIR OWN BATTLES
AND DEMAND UNDERSTANDING. .

CONTENTS

"Firstly you see it, secondly you notice it works and thirdly you start to feel it. After that, everything changes"

Noah Anonis

ACKNOWLEDGMENTS

To those people who kept me going, those people
who kept me alive and those who showed me love,
fun, energy and light.
They know who they are.

1
DOUBT

"Just leave me alone, I need some time to work on my self-doubt."

"Fear and doubt are the same species - but with different spots"

"Doubt if you must. Doubt fantasy, doubt whatever that has no proof. But you must force yourself to never doubt yourself."

"It seems that when I was full of doubt about everything, I believed in nothing and no one. Then I managed to the conquer the doubt and everything was the opposite for some reason!"

"I became so good at doubting myself that I even doubted I was any good at that!"

"There is nothing I can think of that does not have at least a drizzle of doubt, but I am in charge and therefore it was me who decided to doubt doubt itself"

"It was all going so well when I listened to the enthusiastic light, why did I ever let the darkness of doubt in?"

"When it comes to doubt, you must remember it's a very close relative of negativity"

"At one point, I decided to just run with the doubt, to always doubt everything and at least I'd be right when it didn't work out."

"Remember that doubt is only belief turned upside down and inside out."

"I think some doubt comes hand in hand with intelligence and experience – however the really smart thing to do is not to let it lead the way"

"Doubt yourself, then doubt yourself some more and lets see where that gets you!"

"Remember that doubt is rarely helpful and is the enemy of enthusiasm."

"I could decide to make a fantasy of fantastic light and hope just whilst I sit here or I could just sit here and just doubt everything with exactly the same ingredients."

"The diseased doubters will always be there whatever you do. This disease of doubt they will try to pass on to you"

"Where did this doubt suddenly manifest itself and who was it who invented this doubt? Oh yes, that's right – I did"

"They say when in doubt don't. But when in doubt, why not evaluate the situation first with the facts and then I don't doubt that you will make the right choice."

"When I look back, I was beaten as soon as I opened the door to doubt, how I wish I'd opened the door to belief instead."

"They said they did not doubt me but they never believed in me either – to me that's still doubt."

"Doubt – don't talk to me about doubt. It's a pointless exercise."

"I never worry about doubt – because I wait for the proof and then I find there is no room for doubt anyway"

"It was to be a marvelous love affair between enthusiasm and positivity but the third party of doubt came in from nowhere to spoil it."

"The fragility of doubt is like glass if you have the hammer of belief."

"I doubt this is going to work, it's going to be tough, - but hey let's ignore the doubt – what a journey we'll have getting to where we end up."

"In my experience, the doubters even doubt they ever doubted me - once I'd done it of course."

"It's making me almost paranoid, I mean like everything I try and do doubt is there and it stops me — is it following me or am I following it?"

"If you find yourself under the cloud of doubt, take a breath in positivity and breathe out the negativity of doubt."

"Doubt will create imaginary enemies and have you doubting your own shadow if you let it in."

2
PERSPECTIVE

"Sometimes the only thing I had left was to try and find a better perspective – so I kept searching and trying to find that"

"Everything they had, I had more of – yet they always seemed happier. It was almost like they had a better outlook or a better perspective – or something like that!"

"Living in a mental hell is one thing then I realized with a better perspective I could crawl out and that is quite another"

"With my perspective right, nothing can hurt me."

"Circumstances will always change, I just try and make sure my perspective changes along with them"

"I lost my perspective and that was so difficult to understand, but at least I knew that and that was a good thing – from my perspective."

"They say the water always beats the stone if given enough time, but not when it get really hot – the water goes into thin air and the rock remains."

"My perspective changed when I turned the fakeness of fear into pure enthusiasm."

"I didn't understand the language, not even a word and wondered how I would ever move on. Then I changed my perspective to realize we could all still dance together."

"I thought I'd wait, my perspective on it was bound to change someday – but then I decided life is too short to wait for perspective to come to me"

"I changed my view, changed my perspective, just so to enjoy my work more – suddenly I became much better at my work"

"From your perspective it is serious and from mine it's fun. I used to think it was serious too, I just changed my perspective on it"

"I sat down to gain perspective, tried to be calm and remember that even the greatest buildings are built by one on top of two, one on top of two, one on top of two........."

"Everything has a measure, it is only your perspective of the situation that decides whether you are closer to the problem or closer to the solution"

"I look down on you said the giraffe to the gazelle, I look down on you said the gazelle to the rabbit. What measure are we using asked the whale."

3

JOY &
LAUGHTER

"Joy & Laughter are the best free gift you will ever receive, they are yours to hold onto and protect"

"To see a complete stranger experience joy and laughter should still bring joy to you"

"I've always seen it as my job and part of who I am to spread joy and laughter to people. Is there really a better thing you can do?"

"I have the ability to find the funny in almost anything, most of the time it's been a blessing but sometimes it has put me in big trouble – especially when I've found that funny too!"

"Laughter will heal the mind and Joy will heal the soul. Get as much as you can – you'll feel great."

"Try to find something to laugh at everyday for it's good for your health. If you are struggling to find anything to laugh at — at least laugh at that!"

"I opened my purse and I couldn't find anything that wasn't funny."

"I felt no Joy and I felt no laughter, they lived in a different place than my darkness. I started just to do things that made them happen, the darkness lifted and I realized they were there all along"

"I found out that if I silently wished joy and laughter to everyone I met – it came to me too!"

"Now for the science - laughter is contagious and if you multiply it enough times then it turns into and exactly equals joy"

"It is possible to laugh uncontrollably without really knowing why — just think about that for a moment"

"I'm going to try and laugh one more time than I did yesterday. Repeat to fade."

"They made me promise to be serious, but even that made me laugh"

"Smiling has it's place and is a great thing to see on someone's face. Laughter though, you can even feel in another"

"I do try not to laugh when I'm telling a joke, but I've heard it before and it is funny"

"When you have experienced being truly sad, then you will add ten times the value to laughter."

"If you find someone you can laugh together with, even at the tiniest things – keep hold of them for both your sakes!"

"Love & laugh, if you do nothing else in life – love & laugh."

"Joy can be found when you are grateful for everything you have and everything around you. The next step is your inner joy, to do this you must do what you feel is your inner calling, and then simply do that."

"Joy & laughter are your choice – choose them."

"Who was it who told us life was meant to be all serious — ourselves, circumstances, politicians, the system, etc Whoever it was, don't you listen to them — laugh at them instead"

"The best medicine is laughing we get told — so take more medicine"

"I wish artists, musicians and comedians ruled the world and made the rules – surely the world would be a better place"

4
FRIENDSHIP

"My friendship with you is something I never want to lose. I wanted you to know that just in case I don't say it often enough."

"A true friend will always be a true friend, even through the disagreements, the harsh realities and the pain. They won't leave though, for when things get difficult they will still be your true friend."

"Good friends know, they know, you know. You both know. The End."

"When the friends leave because things have gone wrong for you, when they stop calling because your circumstances were too much for them, when it seems no one is around to care – know they were never friends."

"Even with friends, the actions will still speak louder than words."

"Many people go through life without ever having a true friend. I am not one of those people, thanks to you."

"I don't think I can ever match up to the wonderful friend that you are, but I'm sure going to try to."

"You can spend hours talking and listening with someone trying to explain – but your best friend will know and understand it all even before you've uttered a word."

"Great friendship is something that is always made out of choice – on both sides"

"There are two types of close friendship and they are very different. One so solid like huge mountain and will never move and the other is constantly moving, changing but challenging anything in its way like a hurricane"

"A new spark, a certain energy happens when a new friend is made, you know from that moment when you click together and know it will never be broken"

"No one can be friends with everyone and it's a good thing —you'd never be able to fit them all in"

"You say you've no real friends and don't really know how to get friends – two tips, don't look for one and the second is to start by being one."

"There is an unwritten magic when two friends laugh together at a private joke"

"To have a friend that you always see the funny side together but can only hold a serious conversation for five minutes at a time is so special, it would cost millions if it could be bottled."

"If you have to ask yourself the question whether someone is a true friend — just by asking it to yourself also answers it"

"It's easy to keep acquaintances and you can have many who you value. Friendship is when you can tell each other anything and you are still friends despite it!"

"To meet a great friend again after years of absence is like finding those old slippers you thought you'd lost"

"I had no other reason to stand by them, they'd done wrong, they'd made mistakes and they knew that they did. They did not need me to tell them that, I stood by them with the only reason because I was and still am their true friend"

5
INSPIRATION & ENTHUSIASM

"If you can't find the inspiration or the enthusiasm, check all the drawers and all the cupboards and see if it's in there. If not, then you're going to have to look inside you"

"You spend so much time telling me how you can't find the enthusiasm and yet you're so enthusiastic about telling me that!"

"Then all of a sudden I noticed it – maybe the last four letters of the word enthusiasm were giving me a clue – I Am Sold Myself."

"No one is coming on a white horse, no one is coming from the sky either, no one is going to inject you with enthusiasm. Somehow, someway it is going to have to be you."

"When I started accepting that I could make enthusiasm myself – it was a new world."

"It took me years to realize that over half the task was already done just with my enthusiasm for it. If I'd known and acted on that information before – I'd have done so much more."

"I'm not a dancer, I very rarely dance. But when I hear the right music all of a sudden I am enthused, I feel like I'm capable of dancing in the rain!"

"You say that you haven't got much eh – well just use what you've have got then"

"You keep telling me you want to find yourself. Well, you are a blank canvas – so work on creating yourself first and then you'll be much easier to find!"

"The biggest battles you will overcome will double your enthusiasm for life when you've done them against all the odds – it will create a new you."

"You'll soon become an inspiration to others when you tell your story of how you did it and a giver of natural enthusiasm to others."

"I just want to get through this, I can fight my way through with my energy and enthusiasm alone – If I fall and I may, I will get up again and I have to tell myself I can do it."

"Enthusiasm comes in tiny spells, You know you have to strike like a cobra does to a mouse to catch it. Then grab it, take it in and act right away."

"The initial enthusiasm is only the start, it is keeping that same level of enthusiasm throughout that is more difficult"

"I suppose the real talent is not being enthusiastic about something you like to do — that should be easy. The real talent is being enthusiastic for something you don't want to do — but you will."

"If enthusiasm has a colour — it must be yellow or at least bright, it certainly isn't dark."

"I wish I could teach or show you the dark places I have been, until you could actually feel them — you could be nothing but enthusiastic after that."

"I am so tired, my battery is flat, I can't move, I feel like a lead weight, I can't even think. I am going to have one last try – but my best try ever."

"When I look at nature and I see the perseverance of animals who time and again keep going with the very same enthusiasm of their first time I am in awe. I am so in awe that I get embarrassed that I didn't give it all I had."

6
SUCCESS

"Success is a measure, a personal measure. My walking just two steps may be a bigger success than your two hundred miles."

"Successful people all seem to have a few things in common, things like tenacity, belief and courage."

"Maybe it's just simple mathematics and that positive thinking plus positive actions leads to progress which when it is multiplied is success."

"It shouldn't be so surprising how often the most successful want others to join them. They generally want the best for others too."

"Preparation and Information on what you need to do, it will already put you on the road to success."

"Speak to the real successes, and ask them and they'll tell you that they've learnt much more through failure than anything else."

--

It is much simpler and easier to be successful if you can find out what needs to be done and what you need to do first."

"If you are of sound mind and of sound body, you alone are responsible for your success and nothing else."

"Is to aim high but to just fall short less of a success than aiming low but achieving it?"

"My idea of success has changed dramatically over time, these days it's contentment and peace."

"When you wake up in the morning, already know that is success, for some don't."

"When it's the day to be enthusiastic – it's going to be you're lucky day too."

"We must be guarded against the people who point you to the success in any battle, when they have not faced it themselves."

"What is true success? Making a positive difference to even one person and sleeping with a sound mind, should be enough for most."

"Looking at yourself in the mirror, knowing what you've been through and smiling — that's success."

"If you really want to be a success, first you'll need two things — 1 — make a start and 2 — be prepared to fall many times along the way."

"If you take perspective &
enthusiasm and add them
to tenacity & strength the
end will result will be
success, it can be no other
way."

"The enthusiasm you have
nurtured and grown is
now have is a gift to share
to show others the way."

7
DEPRESSION & ANXIETY.

"The only way to explain to some people who don't understand depression would be to ask them to turn wine into water. They'd say it's impossible, yes I'd say, like turning death into life — well I've done that!"

"The pain of depression cannot be translated to those who don't speak depression – let's hope they never have to learn."

"Animals get depressed too, and if you don't believe that just put a tiger in a small cage for a while."

"Depression sufferers don't fear hell. There is every chance they will be looking forward to the trip."

"Even when I feel slightly better I always have death as my insurance policy for happiness, surely that can't be right?"

"I don't understand how people can be smiling — can't they see how I feel?"

"Depression, me? Huh, I used to say. A sign of weakness I would say. They need to be stronger I'd say. Then, when it happened to me I said all those things to myself and none of them worked. It was only then I understood."

"Frightened, scared, panicky, tense, petrified, worried, sad, shaky, jumpy, devastated and terror struck. That's how I feel, but you know what that's not the worse thing – the worse thing is not knowing why."

"If I could just have one big hug and feel loved, but I won't let anyone near me to do it."

"I battle every minute of every hour of every day just to feel like a normal person again— but you won't ever know that."

"I've been told that if I look at it logically then I'll find the direction and the way out of this. But the ones that tell me that don't know the way either."

"They say that you have to go through difficult times to get the good times. Wow, I must be in for a fantastic time anytime soon."

"They told me I was too intellectual and too articulate to be depressed and suicidal. How dare they – I'll show them, they'll be sorry!"

"You can't sleep, you can't stop worrying, you don't want to see people, you can't go out, you don't want to do anything, you have horrible thoughts, you think you are failure, you think about death all the time, you doubt everyone, you think it's all your fault, you must be weak. Oh, and you ask me how I am and I'll say "Fine, how are you.""

"Once I started to get better I vowed to take more chances, play more, take risks, travel more, tell people I love them more. Please let me get better soon."

"I remember thinking if the end of the world came, everyone would be devastated and panic – but they'd only feel like I felt all the time."

"I will never forget how it feels, it was the toughest thing I've ever done. There were many times I thought I'd never be better. I just did everything I could in the end to love and help me. It slowly started to work."

8
HOPE

"I started to realize that hope was important, if I could only find it. I did eventually, but only after I started to hope that I could find a way to hope."

"Hope — people dismiss it, they say you need something more tangible, substantial or a better aim. They are wrong, It's impossible without hope, for hope is the birth of enthusiasm, positivity and then action."

"You can of course have one hope, but why not spoil yourself and have four or five."

"One good thing to remember when it comes to hoping is none of us know what will happen in the future, therefore hopes for the future are always available so grab some of them, hold them and never lose them."

"HOPE – Hang On Pilot Energy, don't leave without me!"

"The agony is real, the difficulty is real, the feeling alone is real, the distance is real but it can all start to subside when you finally realize that the hope is real too."

"Hope alone has saved many lives, it will continue to and that then will lead to great things."

"Hope is not dreaming, they are different - hope is more attached to a sort of loose expectation and dreaming is more of a wish. Hope does have some solidity to it and few realize that."

"Dear Hope - I do hope you understand that I will not get through this without you."

"Muster all your energy to create hope, this will be the best weapon you could ever have to override and conquer fear."

"When your back is against the wall and you can go back no further, when you are so down you can get no lower – it is then you seek and find hope."

"If you can keep dreams and hopes alive they'll do the same for you."

"If your only hope is that — it can't get any worse, then it can only get better. Hope will be there to show you how it can and will get better."

"Hope can come from the tiniest moments — your job is to look for them."

"I started to hope and then things changed, then I dared myself to dream. That is how the new beginning started."

"If there's the tiniest chance it can, the tiniest you can ever imagine – it means it's still possible – that's hope."

"They are the ones who should go down in history, they are the true heroes, the ones who can find hope against the seemingly impossible."

"Pick future events, dates and target them. Hope for them, look forward to them."

"The door to the future is there to be opened with the magic key of hope. You do hold that key."

"In the rain, we can hope for the sun, it may rain a long time – longer than we ever thought possible but the sun will come in time."

"Things aren't going the way I'd hoped they would. I guess I am just going to have to hope some more. And maybe some more after that too"

"Hope that when things get tough you'll always be able to find a way to change your attitude."

"I refuse to abandon hope,
not over this, not over
anything."

9
THE
WINNING
MIND

"The winning mind was trained, worked at and perfected by its owner. Before that, it was just a mind."

"I was in charge of how my mind thought, not the other way around. Wow - that took me a long time to learn."

"I realized everything I did was a success, at the very least I always knew that I would learn something no matter what I did - that is the attitude of the winning mind."

"M.I.N.D. – My Independent Negativity Destroyer."

"I spent so long training my mind to look for the negative, I did not believe you could train it to look for the positive."

"It's a funny thing with the Universe and winning minds, they seem to attract more luck too – like a magnet. Yet, the irony of the losing mind that needs the luck,
gets deserted."

"When you've got a winning mind you are very aware you have it after all you made it."

"The switch from having a losing mind to a winning mind seems a far distance away and hard to achieve to that of the losing mind. However, the winning mind is very aware of the losing mind and how dangerously close it is."

"You have the choice to be stressed with a losing mind or grateful with a winning mind."

"I knew where I had to get to, how to get there was more difficult. I started at the beginning, it was the best place to start, I knew that much – I had to find my winning mind."

"Almost losing my mind was the gateway to finding my winning mind, I still believe that today."

"Keeping your mind on a tight lead is not an easy thing to do, you must first try to stop from wandering then gradually to bring it to heel – it's easier to handle then."

"If I searched hard enough, deep enough, I knew (despite what my losing mind was trying to tell me) that I could find

my winning mind."
"I had kept feeding my mind a losing mentality and it was a losing mind, now imagine my surprise at the results when I fed it the opposite."

"The winning mind knows much, it's tasted bitterness before and fears nothing except one thing — letting the losing mind in again."

"It took me what seemed like an age before I could thank my old losing mind for the wonderful present of my winning mind."

"I have still never met the person with a winning mind that did not work very hard to get it."

"The winning mind doesn't mean I win every single time – it's just an attitude adjustment to give me every chance of doing it"

"I referred to it as my losing mind for so long, on reflection there must have been some winning mind in there all along"

"I was terrified of my mind for believing what it did – as it seemed I was in the always in the dark to why that was– and I never had liked the cold dark, I had always preferred the warm light – so I moved my mind closer to it"

10

ENERGY & INTUITION

"I spotted a pattern quite early on, when I read positive stories or quotes that I could relate to, then I felt a positive energy was starting to connect to it"

"This Intuition, gut feeling is there and yet I had somehow taught myself to doubt it, even though it has proved itself correct to me time and time again"

"Just because science has not yet fully proved the existence of intuition, it does not mean that the day won't come"

" If you feel this clean intuition and energy then surely you must let it flow through you and follow it."

"I only had ever really believed things I could prove. It was everything I was against, to believe in something I couldn't see or hear – but I felt it – oh wow – I felt it."

"Was it a sixth sense, a third eye? That was ridiculous to me, perhaps it still is, but in the end I decided it I did not need to give it an exact label — who for? I just call it energy, the Universe or intuition these days."

"Energy is still the most spoken language and yet still largely the most ignored."

"Obviously some people feel this energy more than others – almost animal like. Maybe they are more in touch with our natural Universe?"

"I believe it and yet I can't prove it to you, I can't show it to you, In fact I know little about it, except I know it is there."

"Imagine the sheer hell of mentally demanding proof to believe in anything, suffering from anxiety being fearful of your own shadow, having depression feeling worthless and doubting everything, but also feeling intuition is correct and all at the same time!"

"It can only be energy, energy is certainly there, all around us – whether we trust ourselves to feel it is another issue, it matters not a jot though if you do or you don't, it is still there"

"You are told and shown your energy must be tense. It's not true, our energy is naturally relaxed"

"In time I noticed that when I was tired or depressed my intuition seemed fuzzily inaccurate and I learnt not to act on it, but when I was fine and in sync – it was always correct"

"Strange that animals rely almost solely on energy and intuition. We are animals too, but we don't"

"The start of some sort of intellectual enlightenment came when I made the connection. Someone belly laughed in company, other people started to laugh too — even though they had no idea what was so funny — they didn't even speak the same language so it was clearly contagious."

- - -

"I don't think that energy and intuition is something we humans need to learn, for I fear through generations we've somehow sadly unlearnt it"

"It's no coincidence that when you tell someone they look good, they are good and their mood improves. The reverse is also true."

"The next thing I spotted was the realization that some were so at home recharging their battery through their moaning, anxieties, negative vibes, worries and cynicism and enjoyed doing it so much, that they almost survived on it and so much so that it gave them a positive energy!"

"The intuition and the energy could only be truthful if it was pure – uninfluenced by human ideas, darkness or lies"

"I'm not suggesting that we need to just rely on intuition or energy and nothing else. I am merely reminding you to give it at least as much credence as you do to the other senses"

"What we believe to be our 'oh so clever human knowledge' has taken the wrong turn somewhere in the past. We talk of our great knowledge of geography yet know little of our own oceans, we talk of our great knowledge of history but learn little from it and the intuition of the wolf we dismiss"

"Energy, it's all energy. Everything is energy, you are energy. The real beauty is the you are in charge of your own energy and you decide what to do with it"

"We come from energy, the sun is energy, the energy will go on forever, it will always shine on"

"You must find the ways to relax to help your own energy, search inside yourself. It will do what you tell it to do, once you find it"

"The borders were created by humans – they don't really exist, separatism and tribalism were human ideas too, look to nature for your answers – for you are nature"

"Let go of the things you don't really need and your energy will grow and grow"

"Energy will make more energy and it will go on until you need to rest, then you must rest and your energy will grow again as you rest"

If you throw all your energy into something you like, that excites you, that becomes a passion then you will follow it as if you are part of it – and you are! "

Noah Anonis is the nom de plume author of the
Free, Sex & Guaranteed Trilogy:
Book 1 – The Manual.
Book 2 – The Enlightenment.
Book 3 – Empowerment.

www.noahanonis.com
noah anonis official fan club.